HOW TO MAKE HIM BURN WITH DESIRE...ONLY FOR YOU

By: **Lanie Stevens**

http://laniestevens.com

Table of Contents

Chapter 1: How to Seduce Him Without Lifting a Finger

Your Energy Is the Ultimate Turn-On

There's a moment—right before a man falls in love—when he feels something he can't explain. He doesn't know where it came from. It's not her smile. Not her voice. Not even the last time he saw her. It's something deeper. Untraceable. A magnetic heat that lives in his chest and spreads to his gut, leaving him unable to focus on anything but her.

That moment doesn't happen by accident.

And you're about to learn how to create it—on purpose.

Remote seduction isn't a trick. It's not manipulation. And it's not about looking hot on social media or playing text message games to get his attention. This is something entirely different.

This is about influence. Invisible, undeniable influence.

You don't have to be in the same room with a man to make his body respond to you. You don't even have to speak. In fact, the most powerful seduction happens in silence. Because when you know how to direct your energy—when you learn how to project emotional sensation into his subconscious—you don't need perfect timing or the right words. You become the moment. The craving. The obsession.

Your energy does what no filter, no push-up bra, and no dirty text ever could.

You create the imprint before he even realizes he's thinking about you.

In this book, you're going to learn how to use Remote Seduction—the art of slipping into a man's subconscious, igniting craving inside his body, and making him see you as the source of his deepest pleasure. You'll learn how to create desire from across the room—or across the world. How to make him feel you emotionally, physically, and sexually—even without a word or a glance. How to implant yourself inside his mind so deeply that no other woman stands a chance.

And you'll do it without ever feeling desperate, needy, or second-best again.

You might be tempted to skip ahead to the "fun part"—the step-by-step technique. Don't. Understanding how and why this works makes you unstoppable. It turns you from a beginner into a goddess. We'll talk about thought projection, quantum entanglement, energy transference, and the psychology behind subconscious craving. It's not just "woo-woo"—it's magnetic science meets feminine power.

And if you think I'm exaggerating, let me tell you a true story.

I have a family member—and I say this with love—who could stop traffic. Not because she's gorgeous. Because people would literally stop and stare, wondering what on earth they were looking at.

She's about five feet tall, built like a fire hydrant, and shaped like a baked potato in orthopedic shoes. Her skin is unpredictable, her eyes are small and suspicious, and her hair looks like a broom that's been through war. Add in teeth that could bite through metal and a voice like gravel—well, you get the picture.

And her personality? She wasn't winning any "most approachable" awards. Let's just say if sarcasm were a perfume, she'd be marinated in it.

By all traditional standards, she should have been invisible to men. Or at best, pitied.

And yet—men obsessed over her. Fought over her. Proposed to her.

She's been married seven times. And every single one of those men? Better-looking. More successful. More charming than she ever should've landed on paper. These weren't desperate men. They were competitive, confident, and totally whipped. They were jealous of her. Afraid to lose her. They orbited her like moons around a planet, completely unaware that they had been seduced at a level far deeper than looks or logic.

How?

Because I taught her. I taught her this Remote Seduction technique. I showed her how to project craving into a man's subconscious so precisely that he didn't even realize what hit him. She became a master. And she used it unapologetically.

She didn't diet. She didn't get a makeover. She didn't "work on herself" in the way women are constantly told to. She just shifted her energy—and the world responded.

If she can do it, you have no excuse.

This isn't about looks. It's not about age. It's not about playing games. This is about emotional energy—transmitted remotely and felt deep inside a man's nervous system. And every woman, including you, has the ability to use it.

Another woman I coached—we'll call her Mia—had been seeing a guy who suddenly disappeared. No warning. No explanation. Just silence.

Instead of chasing him or demanding closure, she decided to try something different. She followed the technique I gave her: she relaxed her body, dropped into a slow, steady brainwave state, and projected specific emotions into his mind—warmth, desire, longing. She didn't think about him. She thought *into* him. She imagined him missing her touch, hearing her laugh, and feeling pulled toward her without knowing why. She imagined intimacy in great detail and it felt so strong that she got excited herself.

For two weeks: silence.

Then out of nowhere, he messaged her.

"You just popped into my head. I couldn't stop thinking about you. I even smelled your perfume this morning, and it drove me crazy. Are you doing something to me?"

She smiled. "Maybe."

Was it coincidence? Not even close.

He felt her because she made sure he did.

You're going to learn how to send that sensation straight into him. How to imprint yourself so deeply into his subconscious that you become his safe place and his fantasy. The one who makes him feel more like a man. The one who turns him on just by existing in his mental space.

And the best part? You don't have to "hope" it works. This is not a fingers-crossed love spell. (Although my love spell is truly magic, too.) It's a real, trainable technique. A woman using it intentionally becomes magnetic—sometimes instantly.

I've seen women use this and get a response from a man who hadn't texted in six months. I've seen a husband who hadn't touched his wife in over a year suddenly start bringing her wine and running her bath. I've seen full-blown reunions between exes who swore it was "really over."

Because when energy is focused, clean, and emotionally charged—it moves people. It pierces right through resistance and cuts to the part of the mind that makes decisions. Especially decisions about love, sex, and intimacy.

So no, this book isn't about how to flip your hair, pose for thirst traps, or send the perfect emoji.

This is about remote arousal. Remote emotional imprinting. Remote magnetic influence.

And once you learn it, you'll never chase again.

Chapter 2: Mind to Body: Making Him Feel You Anywhere

How to Send Desire Straight Into His Skin

Sexual energy is the most powerful creative force in your body. Not because of what it *does*—but because of what it *awakens*. When it's activated with intention, it doesn't stay locked inside you. It moves. It expands. It vibrates outward in waves that can be felt—across rooms, across cities, even across years.

Tantric teachings have always known this. Long before neuroscience and bioenergetics caught up, ancient lovers were working with energy—not just bodies—to stir ecstasy in one another. Tantra teaches that sexual energy isn't just about climax. It's about life force. It's raw feminine power, coiled at the base of your spine, waiting to rise, build, and flood your system—not just for release, but for transmission.

That's the secret most women were never taught: You can send this energy. You can direct it—into a specific man. His body doesn't need to be present. His skin doesn't need to be close. Because what you're stimulating isn't just his body. You're stimulating the receptors in his nervous system that recognize emotional memory, sexual charge, and subconscious desire.

Modern science is just starting to understand how arousal works through the brain-body connection. It's not visual. It's not logical. It's felt. The brain responds to sensation—real or imagined—as if it's happening now. The more emotionally charged the visualization, the more physical the response. You're not just creating a fantasy. You're programming a sensation into his body.

So when you drop into a relaxed, sensual state… when you start breathing as if you're already being touched… when you let energy rise from your core and project it toward him—not just imagining, but *transmitting*—you're lighting up his system in ways he doesn't even understand. He just knows he's turned on. He just knows he can't stop thinking about you. And if he's energetically open, his body will respond. Sometimes instantly.

It started as an experiment. I wasn't trying to fall in love, or even get turned on. I was just playing with energy.

I had a friend back then—let's call him Drew—who lived in another state. He wasn't the kind of man I'd usually go for. We weren't flirty, we didn't talk daily, and we certainly weren't in a relationship. But we had this strange mental chemistry. He was game for anything involving energy, telepathy, or sexuality, and I had started to explore something that would later evolve into the technique I now teach women around the world.

At first, it was curiosity. What happens if I think into him sexually? What happens if I send not just a thought—but a *feeling*—into his body? I didn't picture him. I didn't text him. I didn't even tell him. I just closed my eyes, slowed my breath, and imagined warmth and heat radiating outward from my own body—

searching for his. I pictured him feeling it. I pictured his chest tightening, his pulse racing, his skin responding without knowing why.

And to my shock... he did.

He'd call me hours later, almost breathless. "Did you do something? I felt you. I could swear you touched me. I've been hard all day and I can't stop thinking about you. What are you doing to me?"

We had never kissed. Not even once. But we began triggering intense physical arousal in each other without a single touch. We'd go days, sometimes weeks, without talking—and then out of nowhere, we'd both feel it. The pull. The heat. The ache.

It wasn't fantasy. It was real. It had texture, sensation, weight. And it completely rewired how I saw connection, attraction, and desire.

That experience became the foundation for what I now teach as Remote Seduction: the modern, precise art of using energy, thought, and emotion to reach into a man's body and trigger intense desire from a distance. The concept itself isn't new—remote arousal has existed in tantric traditions, hypnotic seduction, and even spiritual texts for centuries. But what I discovered was how to make it practical. Repeatable. Laser-focused. I didn't invent the idea. But I did turn it into something women could actually use—whether they're married, long-distance, ghosted, or lying next to someone who's emotionally shut down.

That friend and I were never "together" in the traditional sense. But we were bonded by something most couples never experience: telepathic intimacy. Energetic sex. An invisible cord of desire strong enough to override logic. That kind of connection doesn't just fade. It imprints.

And that's when I realized—this isn't just a "fun" trick or a sensual experiment. It's a *tool*. One that any woman can use to seduce, attract, and emotionally enrapture a man on a level he can't logic his way out of. Because when a man *feels* you in his body without a word or a touch... he starts to wonder what else is possible. And that wonder? That's where obsession is born.

Most people think desire starts with sight. That you need to be near him, touching him, turning him on physically. But that's only one layer of attraction. True, consuming desire—the kind that makes him crave you when you're nowhere near—starts in the *mind*. And sexual energy is one of the most powerful carriers of that signal.

Think of it this way: When you're turned on, your energy shifts. Your body heats. Your breath deepens. Your heart pumps faster. But those aren't just internal sensations—they're *broadcast signals*. Your nervous system is generating electricity. Your heart is pumping out a magnetic field. And your emotions—especially intense ones like sexual desire—are vibrating outward in a wave. They don't stop at your skin.

That wave reaches him.

Even if he's miles away.

Even if he hasn't seen you in weeks.

Even if he's asleep.

When your energy is clear and focused—and emotionally charged with sensual intent—it doesn't just "stay in your head." It *touches him*. On a level he may not consciously understand, but his body responds.

His chest tightens.

His skin tingles.

He gets restless, distracted, suddenly craving something he can't name.

And that's exactly the point. Remote seduction doesn't rely on logic. It bypasses the conscious mind and moves straight into his subconscious—the place where cravings form, where memories stick, and where emotional decisions are made.

That's why this works better than any text, photo, or seductive outfit ever could.

Those things go through the eyes.

This goes through the *body*.

You're not just thinking about him—you're thinking *into* him. You're projecting desire like a current, and his nervous system—wired for sensation—is picking it up whether he realizes it or not.

That's why sexual energy is your most powerful weapon.

It's not loud.

It's not obvious.

It's not desperate.

But it's *felt*.

And once he feels it—really feels it—he'll start to associate that sensation with you. Not just your face or your voice. But your presence. Your pull. Your *energy*.

And that? That's when seduction becomes obsession.

Before you can project desire into someone else's body, you have to activate it in your own. Remote seduction doesn't start with him—it starts with you. You are the source. And if your energy is flat, anxious, or scattered, it won't carry. That's why so many women try to "send" feelings to a man and feel like nothing happens. It's not because the technique doesn't work. It's because the signal was weak.

Think of it like heat. You can't warm another room if there's no fire in yours. You have to let the energy build inside your body until it becomes so magnetic, so sensual, so emotionally charged, that it starts spilling out of you without effort. That's when it moves. That's when it touches him. That's when he jolts awake at 2 a.m., hard and aching, thinking of you for no reason he can explain.

Sexual energy is sacred—and it's physical. You don't have to be moaning or dripping in lingerie. You just have to feel it. Fully. In your breath. In your hips. In your chest. Let it rise inside you like a wave. Let it move through your body—not as a performance, but as a private seduction. You're not doing this *for* him. You're doing it for yourself first. You're allowing your own body to become alive with sensation so the signal you send is real.

This is where tantra and energy work meet. In tantra, arousal isn't something that happens *to* you—it's something you awaken. It's not just physical friction or visual stimulation. It's breath, intention, presence, and movement of energy. You build it slowly, deliberately, letting it pool at your center and then rise like smoke through your chest, your throat, your mind. And when you reach that place—where your whole body is humming, not desperate but open—you become magnetic. That's when you project.

You don't have to be touching yourself. You don't have to be "turned on" in a traditional way. You just have to be present in your body. You have to feel the spark—not fantasize, but actually feel. Even five minutes of this state, held in focused awareness, is more powerful than hours of obsessing, scripting texts, or scrolling through photos of him.

Because in that state, you're not chasing.

You're drawing.

You're not hoping he feels something—you're *sending* it.

And that transmission, when done cleanly and with emotional intensity, reaches him in a way no words ever could.

When you begin playing with this energy—really feeling it, not just thinking about it—you'll notice something strange.

His name will pop into your head right before he texts.

You'll feel warmth in your chest as if someone is thinking about you.

You'll get that tight pull in your gut—a magnetism—as if you're being summoned.

This isn't imagination. It's the current between you.

Because when sexual energy is focused with emotion, intention, and sensation, it doesn't just stay in your body. It imprints. It transmits. It enters his field like a whisper he can't hear, but *feels*. Sometimes as a thought. Sometimes as restlessness. Sometimes as pure, physical heat.

And that's just the beginning.

The deeper layers of remote seduction aren't just about sending energy. They're about building a subconscious link—an invisible thread between you that tightens with every pulse of emotion you direct into him.

It's what makes your presence addictive—even in silence.

In the next chapter, we're going to explore exactly how that link works. Not just through science, but through real stories. Real results. The kind that leave men wide-eyed, obsessed, and unable to shake the feeling that *something about you has changed.*

And it has.

Because you're not just fantasizing anymore.

You're transmitting.

Chapter 3: The Invisible Thread Between Minds

Real Stories, Scientific Proof, and How Telepathy Powers Seduction

Most people assume that thoughts are private. That they stay locked inside the walls of your skull—yours and yours alone. But if you've ever felt someone's gaze from across the room... if you've ever had a sudden, electric thought of someone right before your phone lights up with their name... if you've ever woken up breathless from a dream so vivid it felt like a shared experience— then you already know minds don't work in isolation. They reach. They connect. And when emotion is involved, that connection becomes almost impossible to ignore.

The truth is telepathy isn't reserved for psychics or mystics. It's built into the human experience. Most of us are just so overloaded with noise—screens, stress, expectations—that we've forgotten how to listen. How to receive. But that doesn't mean the connection is gone. In fact, it's more active than you realize. Especially when it comes to intimacy.

Let's start with the simplest example: animals. If you've ever had a dog or cat, you've probably seen their uncanny ability to read your mind. My dog, Lolly, has been doing this since the day I brought her home. I don't have to say a word. I don't even have to move. If I so much as *think* about giving her a bath, she's already halfway under the bed, hiding like I've declared war. No visible signals. No cues. Just thought.

I've tried every trick—changing my internal dialogue, distracting myself, even singing songs in my head to mask the thought. Doesn't matter. She still knows. Every single time. And while that's hilarious, it's also telling. Animals haven't lost their telepathic instincts. They still operate through energetic awareness. They *feel* what we think.

Which begs the question: if your dog can sense your intentions, what do you think happens when a man is emotionally, sexually, or subconsciously entangled with you?

He feels you. Even from a distance.

You don't have to send a message. You don't even have to be in contact. There's an invisible thread between you—and when you activate it, he responds.

Not logically. Not in ways he can explain. But in his body. In his thoughts. In his sudden urge to check in, scroll your feed, or wonder what you're doing at midnight. That thread is very real— and it's one of the most powerful tools of remote seduction.

You don't have to take my word for it. Some of the most profound demonstrations of mind-to-mind connection come from people who were never expected to communicate at all.

There's a groundbreaking series called *The Telepathy Tapes*, which documents the inner world of non-speaking autistic individuals—many of whom were once labeled low-functioning or even cognitively impaired. These assumptions couldn't have been more wrong.

Because once they found a way to express themselves—usually through assisted communication or telepathic dialogue—what emerged was jaw-dropping. They described rich, vivid thoughts. Complex emotions. And more incredibly, a shared mental meeting place they all knew by name: *The Hill.*

Not a metaphor. An actual shared internal landscape where they could meet one another—without speaking, without physical presence, without technology. A place where they laughed, learned, exchanged ideas, and even received messages from beyond this world.

They weren't making it up. Many had never met, and yet they described the exact same space, the same energetic details. Some even reported encounters with ancestors or souls who had passed on—offering comfort, wisdom, and reminders of why they came to Earth in the first place.

To them, telepathy wasn't a party trick. It wasn't fringe. It was natural. Normal. *The original human language.*

And according to them, we've all just forgotten it.

They described it like breathing—something that once came easily to everyone, before we drowned it out with screens, distractions, and the belief that "seeing is believing." But just because we stopped using it doesn't mean we lost it. It's still in us. Still active. Still waiting to be awakened.

It's a muscle. And just like any other, it gets stronger the more you use it.

You don't need to be psychic. You don't need to meditate for three hours a day or wear crystals on your third eye (although I've been known to tape one over my third eye just for fun). You just need a willing heart, a calm mind, and a little bit of focus. Your emotions will do the rest.

And when you start applying this to seduction—especially with someone you already have a bond with—the results can be immediate.

That's the beautiful thing about attraction. It sharpens the signal. When desire enters the picture, your energy gets louder. More magnetic. More memorable. It travels with intention—and lands in his nervous system like a lightning strike.

You're not just hoping he thinks of you. You're *giving him the thought.*

And if that sounds impossible, just wait until you hear what happened when I tested it on someone who didn't believe in any of this at all.

Years ago, I had a male friend I'd known since high school. Totally logical, charming, deeply skeptical, and allergic to anything he couldn't measure with a calculator or see under a microscope. He wasn't into energy work, spirituality, or what he lovingly called my "voodoo mind tricks." But he liked me. And he trusted me enough to play along when I proposed a little experiment.

I asked him to send me a message. Not a text, not a call—just a pure, focused thought. Any time during the evening, whenever he felt like it. I didn't want to know when he was doing it. I wouldn't be checking my phone or trying to "tune in" in a meditative trance. I would simply go about my night as usual—and record anything that stood out.

That evening, at 8:20 PM sharp, I was making tea when a thought burst into my mind, so loud and vivid it made me laugh out loud:

"I doubt this shit is working, but I'm trying anyway."

It wasn't just the words—it was his voice. His dry humor. His slight smirk. The tone was unmistakable.

I grabbed my phone and dialed immediately. When he picked up, I didn't say hello.

"Eight twenty," I said. "You sent me, 'I doubt this shit is working, but I'm trying anyway.'"

Silence.

Then the sound of something crashing.

He had fallen off his chair.

Not only had I received the exact message, at the exact time—he had written it down to the minute, thinking I'd never get it.

That night changed something in him. He didn't become a crystal-carrying energy healer, but he never questioned me again.

Because that moment proved something no book or debate ever could.

Telepathy is real.

And more than that—it's *already* happening. Between friends, between lovers, between anyone who's energetically open. Most people just don't recognize it. They think of someone right before getting a text and call it coincidence. They wake up from a dream about an ex, then bump into him at the store, and chalk it up to fate.

But what if it's neither coincidence nor fate?

What if it's *you*?

What if your thoughts, when emotionally charged, really do ripple out like radio waves—landing not just in his mind, but in his body?

This is the foundation of remote seduction. Not imagination. Not fantasy. *Transmission.* A direct energetic signal, created on purpose, and received beneath the surface.

You're not trying to "get into his head." You're already there.

What you're about to learn is how to speak to him without a sound—and make his body feel it like truth.

Not all telepathic moments feel like lightning bolts. Some arrive softer—through dreams, memories, or a strange ache you can't explain. I saw this most clearly in the last few months of my mother's life.

We began having the same dream.

Night after night, we'd both visit the same house. An old, weathered farmhouse tucked somewhere in a small, historic town in Central Texas. We'd never been there in real life. But in our dreams, we knew the place intimately.

There was a tiny kitchen at the back of the house with rusted fixtures and an old screen door that groaned open on squeaky hinges. A narrow wooden staircase led up to creaky floors and bedrooms with pull-chain lights. I could feel the faded wallpaper under my fingers, see the way sunlight slanted through the front window onto a scratched wooden table. The smell— musty and sweet, like dried lavender and dust—was always the same. And every time I woke up, I carried with me a quiet kind of sadness I couldn't explain.

She had the same dream.

We didn't talk about it much at first—just a mention here or there, until we realized the details were identical. The same floor plan. The same creaking staircase. The same door latch and the same uneasy feeling at dawn. It didn't scare us. It fascinated us. And on some deep level, it comforted us too. Like we were being shown something important. Something we couldn't yet name.

After she passed, the dreams stopped.

But the memory never left.

Years later, completely by chance, I found myself driving through a small town I'd never visited before. It was one of those quiet, blink-and-you-miss-it places off the highway. As I slowed at a stop sign, I saw it.

The house.

Restored now, with fresh paint and a welcoming sign out front—a Bed & Breakfast. But the bones were the same. My heart stopped. I parked and went inside.

The owner was kind and curious. When I described what I remembered, he nodded slowly and said, "You must be remembering it from the war."

He told me that during World War II, the house had been used to house returning military officers. It had gone through years of disrepair before being renovated, but he kept all the original photographs. And when he brought them out, I could hardly breathe.

Every detail matched. The kitchen, the fixtures, the screen door, the staircase. Even the little lightbulbs with pull-chains in the upstairs bedrooms. It wasn't a coincidence.

It was something deeper.

Maybe a past life. Maybe a shared soul memory. Maybe something neither of us will understand until long after we're gone. But it was real. And it taught me something I now know for sure:

The mind isn't locked inside the body. The soul isn't bound by time.

And the connections we feel—especially the ones that defy logic—are often more real than anything we can prove.

When women ask me, "Can he really feel me when I use Remote Seduction? Even if we're not speaking?"

My answer is simple.

You don't need him to understand it.

You just need to remember that *you* already do.

Sexual energy has a way of breaking through where words can't. It moves past logic, past anger, even past heartbreak. It's raw, primal, and sometimes shockingly healing—especially when directed intentionally across distance.

One of my closest friends experienced this in a way that still gives me chills.

She had broken up with her ex months earlier. And to be clear, she *hated* him. Not the polite kind of dislike that fades with time—but a visceral, deep-seated anger. He had treated her terribly, and she wanted nothing to do with him.

But here's the twist: she still missed the sex.

The chemistry between them had been electric. And one day—out of curiosity more than anything—she decided to try something.

She didn't call him. Didn't message. Didn't even post anything suggestive. She simply closed her eyes, relaxed her body, and started using the Remote Seduction technique. She focused on him with precision—not with love, not with longing, but with pure, directed desire.

She imagined him in vivid detail. The smell of his skin. The weight of his hands. The sound of his breath when he was fully immersed in her. She didn't just think about him— she *felt* him. She welcomed him into her mental and physical space and allowed herself to fully surrender to the fantasy.

And what happened next shocked her.

She said it was like he was *there*. Not just emotionally, but physically. His energy was on her bed. On her skin. Inside her. The experience was so vivid, so intensely sensual, she opened her eyes halfway through—genuinely startled by the absence of his body. Her mind and her nervous system were completely convinced he had been in the room.

But that wasn't the strangest part.

Later that same day, he called her.

Not to apologize. Not to rekindle anything. Just to ask something absurdly trivial—about a mutual friend's dog, of all things. But his tone was different. Softer. Curious. Like he was checking to see if the door was open. And for the first time since their breakup, he invited her to lunch. "For old time's sake," he said.

She didn't go. She wasn't interested in reigniting anything with him. But she knew exactly what had happened.

He felt her.

Despite the months of silence, despite the bitterness, despite her very clear boundaries—he felt her sexual energy land inside his system. And it stirred something in him. Something that made him reach out, even without understanding why.

That's what remote seduction does when it's fueled by erotic charge. It slips under defenses. It bypasses anger, ego, and even conscious memory. It touches the deepest, most animal part of the mind—the part that responds to sensation, not reasoning.

And it doesn't require love.

That's the part most people don't understand. You can absolutely feel disgusted by someone—and still imprint them erotically. Sexual energy runs on its own circuitry. It's deeper than personality. Deeper than compatibility. It's pure body-to-body language. And when you speak it fluently, distance becomes irrelevant.

You don't need physical contact to seduce someone.

You need emotional electricity.

You need focus, sensation, and the willingness to project your energy into their space like a heat-seeking pulse.

Because when you do that—when you tune your erotic energy like a frequency and broadcast it into someone's field—they *will* feel it.

They might not know why they're suddenly restless.

They might not understand why they keep thinking of you—or dreaming about you, or checking your old photos, or re-reading texts they swore they deleted.

But their body knows.

Their subconscious knows.

And eventually, the rest of them catches up.

The most overlooked gateway to another person's mind is the one they slip into every night: sleep.

Dreams are not random noise. They're the subconscious in free motion—processing memories, emotions, and impressions it couldn't fully handle while awake. And when someone is asleep, the critical filters of logic, skepticism, and emotional defense are lowered. That's when they're most receptive. Most open. Most easily influenced.

Which means: it's the perfect time for remote seduction.

You don't have to wait for them to be conscious. In fact, sometimes the strongest responses come from seduction done *during* sleep. Not your own—*his*.

Have you ever dreamed about someone you hadn't thought of in years… and suddenly woke up aching for them?

That's no accident.

It could be a memory surfacing—or it could be *them*, reaching out on a non-verbal, subconscious level. Most people write this off as random, but in the world of quantum seduction, it's one of the most fertile grounds for connection.

I've had clients practice remote influence during a man's sleep cycle—usually late at night, right as they know he's winding down or already dozing off—and within days, that man will say something like:

"I had the strangest dream about you."

"You showed up last night... I swear I could smell your perfume."

"Were you thinking about me last night? I couldn't sleep."

These aren't just cute coincidences. They're neurological echoes. The result of subconscious imprinting done at a time when the mind is open and unguarded.

There's a reason dream telepathy studies have shown stronger results than many waking influence experiments. When someone is asleep, their brain drops into deep theta and delta waves—frequencies that are also associated with meditation, hypnosis, and trance states. These states are highly receptive. They allow emotional impressions to embed without resistance.

In the early 1970s, studies by Montague Ullman and Stanley Krippner at the Maimonides Medical Center showed that subjects could transmit images to dreamers with statistically significant accuracy—just by focusing on a picture or idea while the receiver slept.

If *images* could be transmitted that clearly... what about *desire*?

What about seduction?

When you learn how to emotionally charge your energy and beam it into his sleeping field—especially with erotic visualization—it lands in a place where his conscious mind can't rationalize it away. It becomes part of the dream. And dreams, especially the vivid ones, linger in the nervous system long after waking.

He may not remember the details. But he'll remember how he *felt*.

He'll wake up with a craving he can't name.

He'll replay those sensations during the day, reaching for you mentally, not knowing why.

That's how remote seduction slips beneath the surface.

It's not a shout. It's a whisper. A touch that happens in the dark, when no one's looking, and no one's thinking too hard.

You don't need to be in his bed to turn him on.

You just need access to his subconscious.

And when you understand the rhythm of his mind, the softness of his sleep, the vulnerability of his dreams—you can slip in quietly, like silk over skin.

You become the feeling he can't forget.

The image he wakes up missing.

The ache he carries into morning.

This isn't fantasy. It's precision.

And it's only the beginning of what your mind—and your energy—can do.

Sometimes when a woman starts using remote seduction regularly, she'll describe something that sounds almost supernatural.

She'll say things like:

"I swear I felt him touch me."

"My body reacted before I even knew what I was doing."

"I was just lying in bed and suddenly got flushed—like someone was watching me... and I liked it."

These aren't delusions. They're phantom sensations—real physical responses triggered by energetic presence. The body remembers. The nervous system stores everything. And when you've shared intimacy with someone—or even deeply fantasized about it—those patterns don't just disappear. They linger like a scent on a pillow. Like heat left in the sheets after someone gets up.

There's a term in somatic therapy called *body memory*. It refers to the way your nervous system stores emotion and touch, especially when those experiences were intense. That means every sigh, every whisper, every skin-on-skin sensation is *encoded*. And when you begin to focus your energy back on that person— especially during remote seduction rituals—you start to light up those dormant circuits.

But here's the twist: it's not just happening in your body. It's happening in *his*.

Your energetic projection becomes a kind of psychic foreplay. You're not in the room, but your presence is. You're not touching him, but his body reacts. The heart races. The breath quickens. Sometimes, the arousal is so strong he thinks it's spontaneous. Or he'll assume he just had a "dirty dream" or an unexplained urge to call you, touch himself, or see you again.

He doesn't realize you've already touched him—with thought.

And because male arousal is so physical, so body-driven, the imprint of that sensation hits fast and lingers long. Especially when it's tied to emotion.

This is why *repetition* matters in remote seduction.

Each time you send that charge; you deepen the anchor. You condition his body to crave you—just like a habit. Just like an addiction. Not with logic. Not with words. But with *feeling*.

The more he feels you, the more his subconscious associates pleasure with your presence—even when you're not physically present. You become the drug. The trigger. The reward.

This is also why men often dream about you after a strong session.

You'll wake up from a vivid fantasy and hours later he'll text, "I had the craziest dream about you."

Or he'll say, "You randomly popped into my head while I was in the shower." Or even admit, "I felt you last night. I don't know how to explain it, but I felt you."

They'll shrug it off as weird. You'll know better.

Because remote seduction, done right, creates echoes. Emotional fingerprints. And those fingerprints stay on his skin, long after the energy is sent.

Let me tell you a story I've never shared publicly—not in a book, not on a podcast, not even with most close friends. Partly because I was afraid no one would believe me. And partly because I didn't want to speak his name into the open. And partly because I was afraid someone would knock on my door. Not in a good way.

I once dated a man who worked for a three-letter agency. A high-ranking member. I won't say which agency, and I won't share what he told me, because some things still don't feel safe to put in print. But I will tell you this: he had abilities. The kind you read about in classified documents. The kind most people think are fiction.

We never talked about remote seduction. In fact, I never told him what I was capable of. I didn't want to. I knew enough about his world to know I didn't want to engage in that kind of energetic vulnerability with him.

Still, there was a strange chemistry between us. A charged tension I didn't quite understand. We weren't even intimate. Never had sex. Never so much as kissed. But one night, we were on the phone, having a completely ordinary conversation—no flirting, no buildup, nothing sexual at all—and suddenly I *felt* something.

A hand. On my body. Not in my mind. *On* me.

Specifically, I felt his hand between my legs. The exact sensation. As if he were physically touching me.

I gasped.

And before I could say a word, he said, calmly, "Did you feel that?"

I was stunned. My entire body froze. This wasn't visualization. This wasn't energetic flirtation. This was actual sensation—and it crossed a boundary I hadn't agreed to. I hadn't even been thinking about him in that way.

I didn't say "lose my number," but part of me wanted to.

A few weeks later, I was cleaning my house when I felt it again—that jolt of awareness, like someone was watching me. Only stronger. The energy was so intense it stopped me in my tracks. I knew he was outside. I didn't see him. I just *knew*.

I picked up the phone and called him.

"Where are you?" I asked.

"I'm home," he said.

"No," I said. "You're in visitor parking. Right in front of my house."

He was silent.

"You're not even in your Lexus. You're in a truck."

More silence. Then, finally: "Yes."

He didn't even live in my city. He lived seventy-five miles away. And yet he had driven all that way—not to knock on my door, not to talk to me—but just to sit outside and *be* in my field.

To feel me. To connect to my energy in a way that bypassed every physical barrier.

It was the last time I ever spoke to him.

I blocked his number. But more importantly, I blocked him energetically. I shut every channel. Cut every cord. Sealed every entry point in my field. And I never heard from him again.

Why am I telling you this?

Because I want you to understand how *real* this is. Remote energy can be used to seduce, to comfort, to love—but it can also be misused. And the more sensitive you become, the more you need to learn how to protect your field.

The good news? He told me something in that moment I'll never forget.

He said, "What I can do, you can do. If you ever wanted to."

That was the gift.

Because what you're learning in this book isn't make-believe. It's not theory. It's not "woo." It's real. And powerful. And yes—if you want it—it's yours.

Chapter 4: Turning Fantasy Into Need

Creating Cravings He Can't Escape

There's a moment during remote seduction when the body begins to blur the line between imagination and experience. Your breath catches, your chest flushes, and for a second, your hands tremble like they've been touched—when they haven't. Your brain, flooded with arousal and mental imagery, doesn't know the difference. It only knows what you feed it.

And when what you feed it is vivid, focused, and emotionally charged, it begins to respond as if the scene is real. But here's the most delicious part: his body responds too.

It doesn't matter whether he's lying in bed across town or sitting in a meeting halfway across the world. The subconscious speaks a universal language—one that travels across time zones, relationship labels, and even memory. When you infuse your vision with erotic energy and direct it with emotional precision, your fantasy becomes a tether. A sensory thread that wraps around him and whispers, *Come closer. You want this. You want me.*

He might not understand it. He might chalk it up to a dream, a mood swing, a sudden wave of wanting that came out of nowhere. But his body knows. His body always knows.

This is the moment when fantasy becomes foreplay—and when remote seduction graduates from theory into undeniable reality.

A woman I knew once had a long, beautiful, complicated relationship with a man who broke her heart. He betrayed her, mistreated her, and left a trail of emotional wreckage she swore she'd never forgive. She hated him. Couldn't speak his name without venom. And yet... the sex had been incredible. The connection, at least in that one dimension, was unforgettable.

Months passed after the breakup, and she had no intention of ever speaking to him again. But one night—out of boredom, curiosity, or maybe a mix of revenge and longing—she decided to try remote seduction.

She said she wasn't fantasizing to win him back. She didn't even want to feel affection. She just wanted to know if the connection was still alive on that visceral level. If the tether they once had could still be activated without a word or a touch.

So, she did what I taught her. She dropped into an alpha brainwave state. She slowed her breath. She imagined their old dynamic—not as a memory, but as a current moment. The smell of his skin. The pressure of his body. The sound of him when he wanted her. She imagined the exact moment of surrender—not hers, but his. The moment he couldn't take it anymore. The moment he needed her.

And then, she let it go.

No texts. No contact. Just energy.

A few hours later, her phone lit up. His name appeared. Her stomach dropped.

He didn't say anything dramatic. He didn't confess his love. He asked about something completely irrelevant—an old hoodie, a birthday gift from years ago. But his tone? Different. Kind. Soft. Tentative.

And then he asked, "Would you want to grab lunch sometime? Just to catch up."

She almost laughed out loud. It was the same man, but something in him had shifted. And she knew why.

He felt it.

Even if he didn't understand it, his body had responded to hers. His mind had picked up the signal. And it had compelled him, unconsciously, to seek her out—not for closure, but for reconnection.

When you trigger erotic memory from afar—when you stimulate the emotional parts of the brain responsible for bonding, pleasure, and recall—it acts like a psychic fingerprint. It leaves a trace. Not just of you—but of how he felt around you. Inside you. Because in that moment, whether he admits it or not, he feels *possessed* by something invisible. A desire he can't fully place but can't ignore either.

That is the magic of focused fantasy.

And it's only the beginning.

Every time you engage in fantasy with emotional and physical presence—especially when you're in that slowed-down, sensual, alpha brainwave state—you begin to create what neuroscientists call *an embodied simulation.* You're not just "thinking about" something. You're simulating it in the full theater of your nervous system. The brain's visual cortex, somatosensory pathways, and limbic centers all light up as if the real experience is happening.

And here's the secret no one talks about: when you do this with intention, with arousal, and with emotional focus on a specific person, you're not only lighting up your own body—you're pulling theirs into the simulation too.

This isn't fantasy for entertainment. This is fantasy as energetic activation.

When you close your eyes and feel him responding to you—feel his skin tighten, his heart race, his breath hitch—you're doing more than imagining. You're sending. You're transmitting that signal into the quantum field, and because the mind doesn't exist in isolation, his subconscious picks it up. Especially if you've already had a physical or emotional connection with him before.

The brain is always scanning for familiar emotional patterns. It doesn't care if those signals come from a face-to-face interaction, a dream, or a deeply embodied fantasy. It cares how the signal *feels.* And when that signal is drenched in desire, wrapped in the memory of touch, and carried on the frequency of love or lust? It locks in.

This is how craving is built.

Not through logic. Not through strategy. Through *emotional repetition.* Through sensory seduction. Through the kind of vivid fantasy that doesn't stay in your mind—it lives in your body.

When you do this right, he won't just think of you. He'll feel you. And he won't be able to explain why he suddenly misses you, dreams about you, or wakes up hard and aching without knowing what triggered it.

You triggered it.

And the more you practice, the more undeniable it becomes.

You might wonder, how long does it take? How many times do I have to do this before he feels it?

There's no fixed number—because energy doesn't respond to time. It responds to *intensity.* To clarity. To presence.

One well-executed, emotionally charged projection can reach deeper than weeks of lukewarm thoughts. This is not about effort—it's about *emotional precision.* You don't need to fantasize for hours or repeat scripts like a robot. You need to feel it. To become it. To let your body, your breath, your desire become the transmission.

The truth is, fantasy becomes reality when it's practiced in the body. The more you drop into sensation, into detail, into the truth of your arousal, the more powerfully your energy imprints itself on his subconscious.

And yes—he will respond.

Sometimes it's immediate: a message, a call, a comment that proves he felt it. Other times, it's more subtle—a shift in his mood, a sudden softness in his tone, a strange coincidence that puts him in your orbit again. That's not fate. That's you, rewiring the invisible cords between you with nothing but energy.

You've already done this in your life—probably without realizing it. The sudden urge to check your phone, only to see a message from someone you were thinking about. The flood of emotion that makes your chest ache when someone you love is in pain, even before they tell you. The deep knowing that someone is thinking of you—even when there's no evidence.

You're not imagining these things. You're picking up signals. And now? You're learning how to *send* them.

This chapter was not just about technique. It was about embodiment. Understanding that every fantasy you have holds a seed of reality—if you know how to feed it.

In the next chapter, you'll learn how to make your energy unforgettable. You'll discover how to create an emotional signature inside him that's so compelling, so undeniable, he feels you even when he's with someone else. You'll take what you've learned here—and deepen it into something unbreakable.

You are not just a woman thinking sexy thoughts.

You are a sender.

A seductress.

And you're about to become the craving he can't explain.

.

Chapter 5: The Unbreakable Pull

Entangle Him Energetically—And He'll Always Feel You

Quantum entanglement occurs when two particles become inextricably linked, and whatever happens to one instantly affects the other—no matter how far apart they are.

Einstein famously called it "spooky action at a distance."

Modern physicists have proven it again and again: when two particles become entangled, they no longer behave as independent units. Change one, and the other responds.

Instantly.

Distance doesn't matter. Time doesn't matter. Nothing stands between them.

But this isn't just about particles. It's about people, too. You can become entangled with another human being in countless ways:

Through love.

Through intimacy.

Through a glance across a crowded room.

Through a simple thought.

Sometimes, entanglement is formed by physical touch. Sometimes, it's created simply through focused intention.

I saw this power firsthand when I trained in energy healing with Dr. Eric Pearl in what's called "The Reconnection." We were taught how to tune into unseen frequencies—how to feel them ripple through the air, bend between hands, vibrate inside bodies.

As we practiced, I would hover my hands over another participant, and suddenly, crazy things would happen.

We would feel as if we were floating.

Flying. Spinning together through space — *together*.

No one was touching.

But our energy fields merged.

We were completely entangled.

One movement, one ripple, one breath—and we both felt it instantly.

Later, I learned that you didn't even need hands to project energy. Your eyes alone could send energy surging across space. We practiced projecting healing through nothing but gaze—and the results were mind-blowing.

Hearts raced.

Fields shifted.

Connections sparked like live wires.

That's when I truly understood:

Entanglement is everywhere. It is the natural, invisible glue that binds all things.

You can become entangled with someone simply by thinking about them.

By looking at a photo.

By hearing their name.

During intuitive readings, when clients send me photographs of themselves and their person of interest, I feel it immediately. The moment I look at the image with intention, the bond forms.

It's like slipping inside their energy field, feeling their emotions, their hopes, their unspoken longings.

And sometimes, people feel the pull without ever understanding why.

Once, when I was at a mall with my baby niece—this tiny, beautiful being radiating pure light—a woman approached us. She was admiring the baby, drawn in like a moth to a flame. But then she paused, looking serious, almost reverent.

"I need to touch her," she said. "Do you mind?"

Surprised, I said, "Of course, go ahead."

She gently touched my niece's tiny hand, then smiled and said something I will never forget:

"I had to touch her... or I would have been entangled with her forever."

At the time, I didn't fully understand what she meant. But now?

I know she wasn't being dramatic.

She was speaking truth.

Energy recognizes energy.

Connection is real.

And once you are entangled, you are linked.

This is why remote seduction is not only possible—it's inevitable.

You don't need to be lovers.

You don't even need to have met.

You can create entanglement across space, across time, across every physical limit humans think they have.

Sometimes it happens naturally—an intense moment of eye contact, a brush of fingertips, a long-held gaze across a crowded bar. But sometimes? You can create it intentionally.

Here's how to start weaving the thread:

- If you encounter someone in person, use eye contact. Hold it longer than feels normal. Smile subtly. Let your energy pour through your gaze.

- While looking, mentally send a message: "You feel drawn to me," "You want to know me," or simply "You can't resist me."

- Later, close your eyes and vividly visualize the person— engage all your senses. Imagine their voice, their scent, the texture of their clothing.

- Focus your connection through three points: the third eye (intuition), the throat (communication), and the heart (emotion).

- Let yourself feel as if you already know them intimately, even if you've never spoken a word.

Once entangled, it doesn't matter if days or months pass. It doesn't matter if oceans stretch between you. Your energy will still reach them.

I once locked eyes with a man across a crowded meeting room.

No conversation.

Just a few electric seconds.

Later, I took a few minutes to visualize him—to weave the energy between us, even though I didn't know his name.

Two days later, I ran into him again. Same spark, same magnetic pull.

Still no words.

The third time fate crossed our paths, he came straight to me—drawn by an invisible thread that had been pulling him closer all along. When he spoke, it was with the certainty of a man speaking to someone he already knew.

And in a way, he did.

The spark we had ended up in a long-term friendship. The universe pulled us together based on the power of our encounter and the hidden desire we unknowingly ignited but it wasn't physical.

Because when two energies become entangled, the mind, body, and soul recognize the bond even before the conscious mind can catch up.

Entanglement can be created—but it can also be dissolved. And sometimes, it needs to be.

When connections no longer serve you, when relationships become draining or painful, it's important to unplug those energetic cords.

Here's how:

- Enter a meditative, relaxed state.
- Visualize the person you wish to disconnect from.
- See cords or energetic plugs connecting them to you—especially at the heart, throat, and sexual centers.
- One by one, gently unplug each cord and watch it retract back to them.
- As you remove each cord, imagine that spot filling with radiant golden light, sealing and healing the space.

You'll be amazed at how different you feel afterward—lighter, freer, more fully your own.

Because entanglement is real. It's beautiful when chosen with intention. But it must always be handled with care.

Every thought, every connection, every visualization strengthens the web between you and the one you desire.

Remote seduction works because the connection is already there—or because you are about to create it.

And once the thread is woven, distance will no longer matter.

Desire will no longer be contained. And neither will you.

Some women don't even know they're doing it. Others? They do it on purpose. Let me tell you about a friend of mine who mastered this kind of silent seduction—without ever touching the man.

Some people think entanglement only happens through intense relationships or physical intimacy. But the truth is—it can begin in the blink of an eye.

A friend of mine and I used to go to the same upscale restaurant for live music and appetizers. One night, across the bar, we spotted a man who was, in her words, "a complete snack." I was happily in a relationship with my fiancé at the time, so I didn't give it a second thought. But she—oh, she was curious.

She didn't approach him. Didn't flirt. Didn't even make direct eye contact. She just locked in on him energetically and silently sent a seductive message.

A few minutes later, he blushed. Visibly. Then he shifted in his seat, glanced around like he was trying to shake something off, and kept sneaking glances in our direction. He was flustered—obviously feeling the pull—but he never came over. When he finally left, she smiled and said, "I sent him a message: 'You're going to ask me out.' Guess he wasn't ready."

We laughed it off and figured that was the end of it.

Fast forward a couple of months. Different night. Different restaurant. This time, a place we'd never been before.

And there he was.

Same guy. Across the room again—this time with another woman. My friend did it again. Quietly. Confidently. She sent him the same seductive pulse she had before. And just like before, he flushed, looked rattled, and couldn't stop glancing at her. Still, he didn't act.

We figured it was just another strange coincidence.

But then, it happened.

The next time we saw him—another month later—he made a beeline straight for her. No hesitation.

"It feels like I know you," he said. "I swear we've never spoken, but I remember everything about you. The way you looked. The vibe. It's like I've been trying to figure out how to find you again."

She just smiled and said something vague. He stared at her, a little in awe, and admitted, "I'm embarrassed to say how often I've thought about you. There's something about you I can't explain."

They went on to have a brief fling. Nothing serious. But even after it ended—her choice, by the way—he kept calling every few months, just to check in. No pressure. No drama. Just a man haunted by something he couldn't shake.

And here's the kicker: She's not a conventionally stunning woman. She's attractive, yes—but not someone you'd expect to make a man feel possessed.

It wasn't her appearance that gripped him.

It was her energy. Her focus. Her ability to entangle him without saying a word.

And it worked.

That's the real seduction.

Not in the hips or lips or witty replies—but in the silent, magnetic field you create between you and another person. The one that makes his chest tighten when you walk by. The one that lingers long after the moment is over.

Entanglement isn't just a theory. It's real. It's tangible. And once you understand how to create it, you'll start noticing how often people feel you before they ever *see* you.

Because the moment you weave that energetic thread?

He'll feel the pull.

And he won't even know why.

Chapter 6: Erotic Rewiring

Make Him Crave You Like a Habit He Can't Break

Desire is not an accident. It's a pattern—built, reinforced, and embedded deep within the emotional centers of the brain. When we feel it for someone, especially when it's intense or addictive, it's not just chemistry. It's neurobiology, energy, and memory working together like a perfectly rigged trap, rewiring us from the inside out.

Scientists have long known that the brain stores emotionally charged memories differently than ordinary facts. The areas most responsible for this are the amygdala and the hippocampus. The amygdala tags memories with emotional weight, branding certain moments into your nervous system like fire, while letting others fade away without a trace. The hippocampus, meanwhile, holds the rich, sensory details—the scent of his skin, the sound of his voice, the way the light hit his face when he looked at you with hunger. Together, these two systems form emotional imprints—so vivid, they can trigger full-body responses years after the original experience.

But here's the secret: that imprinting doesn't have to happen by accident. You can create it. You can build it, deliberately and precisely, inside someone else's emotional mind. You don't need fate or chemistry to do it. You can become the source of his craving—through focused thought, sexual energy, and the power of emotional repetition.

That's what erotic rewiring really is. It's not seduction through flirting, or physical appearance, or witty banter. It's seduction through the subconscious. Through memory. Through the addiction pathways in the brain. And the wildest part is this: the brain doesn't know the difference between something real and something vividly imagined—especially when emotion is involved. This is why top athletes mentally rehearse victories, why actors visualize standing ovations, why successful people imagine the future they want until it becomes a reality. The body responds to emotionally charged visualization as if it's really happening. And so does his.

Once you understand this, you stop trying to get his attention with external tactics. You start working where the real power lives—inside his nervous system. The key lies in three elements: visualization, emotion, and repetition. When you imagine him touching you, needing you, losing himself in you— and when you let that fantasy come alive with real breath, real energy, and real desire—you aren't just entertaining a fantasy. You're activating neural pathways. You're triggering dopamine. You're setting off the same chemical systems that drive motivation, craving, and arousal.

And the more often you do it—with clarity, emotion, and sensual focus—the stronger the wiring becomes. Over time, he begins to associate you with a rush of physical sensation, sexual anticipation, and emotional satisfaction. His body starts to expect you. His thoughts drift toward you without warning. He doesn't understand why you keep showing up in his mind—but you do. Over and over again.

This is how people become addicted to one another—not because of looks, or charm, or even compatibility—but because of how they *feel* when they think about the person. You're not seducing his eyes. You're seducing his emotional memory. And once you've planted those associations deep enough, it's very hard for him to walk away.

That's when craving begins. And cravings, by their very nature, seek resolution. They want contact. Closure. A hit of the thing they're wired to want. And you've made yourself that thing—without ever saying a word.

What makes this so much more than "thinking sexy thoughts" is the precision behind it. You're not just fantasizing. You're shaping an entire neurological experience. You're directing desire like an artist with a brush—each stroke purposeful, emotional, alive.

This is what happens when remote seduction is done properly: you don't just make him think about you. You make him *feel* you, physically and emotionally, until his body reacts on instinct. His heart speeds up. His breath shallows. His mind floods with a familiar ache. And all of it—every reaction—gets tied to you.

Even if he's moved on.

Even if he's with someone else.

Even if he thinks he's over you.

Suddenly, you're the thought that won't leave. You're the ghost he can't shake. You're the feeling he can't name—but that he secretly craves.

This isn't magic. It's neuroscience. The male brain is designed to seek novelty, but it's also wired for emotional patterning. When you keep delivering that emotional and sexual energy over and over again, you're reinforcing the neural loop between you and him—one that starts to override everything else.

That's why, one day, he'll hear your name and his chest will tighten. He'll smell something that reminds him of you and feel a pull in his body. He'll be kissing someone else, and suddenly, it won't feel quite right.

Because it's not about logic anymore.

It's about imprinting.

It's about addiction.

Studies on romantic love have shown that it activates the same brain regions as drug addiction. The dopamine system goes wild. The rational part of the brain—the prefrontal cortex—takes a back seat. The brain begins lighting up for cues associated with that person: a word, a song, a memory, a fantasy.

And in this case, *you* are the cue. Your energy. Your memory. Your signature on his nervous system.

Every time you do the technique—every time you project pleasure, connection, erotic presence—his brain reacts. Whether he wants it to or not.

And that's how you become the habit he can't break.

This is why your intention matters. You're not just sending a casual signal into the air. You're entering his emotional system. You're becoming a part of his inner world. When you do this work—especially the erotic kind—you're altering what his mind, body, and heart associate with pleasure, safety, and desire. You're rewiring what turns him on. That's not something to take lightly.

If you do it from a place of obsession or insecurity, the energy becomes muddy—and your results will reflect that. But if you step into it with confidence and clarity, grounded in your own worth, the power you carry becomes magnetic. You're not just making him think of you. You're imprinting him with emotion. You're becoming the one woman who stands out in a sea of forgettable experiences—because you touched him where it mattered most: inside his memory, his nervous system, his subconscious.

One of my former clients understood this perfectly. Her ex had moved away and gotten engaged to someone else. He'd blocked her number, deleted every photo of her from his social media, and seemed to vanish from her life. Most people would've taken that as a hard stop. But not her. She didn't chase. She didn't beg. She simply got quiet... and powerful.

She began doing the techniques from this book—projecting energy through thought, breath, memory, and desire. She didn't send him messages. She didn't try to "manifest" him with vision boards or affirmations. She seduced him the way a master would: energetically, invisibly, through the frequency of her own body.

At first, it was just small shifts. A dream here. A feeling there. Then, without warning, he unblocked her. Reached out. Nothing heavy—just a meme, a song, a random comment. But each message carried weight. He was checking to see if the bond was still alive.

Over time, the emotional energy she'd been sending started to bloom. He confessed that he couldn't stop thinking about her. That he'd dreamt of her nearly every night. That he couldn't touch his fiancée without feeling her absence in the room.

Eventually, he flew across the country just to see her. They didn't sleep together. She didn't need to rush it. The energy was doing everything for her. He sat across from her and said, "I don't know what you did to me... but I can't break it."

And she just smiled—because she knew.

She hadn't manipulated him. She hadn't tricked him. She had simply reactivated everything he once felt and anchored it with erotic charge. She had rewired the memory of her into his emotional and sexual nervous system so deeply that it overrode everything else. And once that wiring is in place, it's nearly impossible to escape. That is the true art of erotic rewiring.

You aren't trying to make someone love you. You're making them feel you—in their skin, in their breath, in the quiet hours of the night when no one else is around. You're becoming the itch they can't scratch. The ghost they can't forget. The craving that won't fade.

Through emotion, through repetition, through the power of your own sensual energy, you're creating a memory loop in his mind—one that always leads back to you.

He might not understand it. He might try to run from it. But in the end, he'll only feel whole when he's with you.

And the best part? You did it all without ever touching him.

You're not just a woman he once knew. You're a sensation his body is still trying to process. When you step into remote seduction with clarity, intention, and emotional precision, you stop being a memory and start becoming a chemical event—an echo in his nervous system, a pattern in his desire. You become the loop he can't escape.

He may believe he's moved on. He may even tell himself he's over you. But his body? His instinct? His need? They know better. Because you didn't just touch his skin—you touched his wiring. And once the imprint is there, it doesn't fade easily. It replays. It pulses. It burns through him at odd hours of the night, when logic is asleep and only the truth remains.

What no one tells you is this: the more confident you become in your power—the more you own the sensual force of your feminine mind—the more undeniable your pull becomes. Remote seduction isn't just about reactivating his desire. It's about activating yours. It's about remembering who you are when you stop waiting to be chosen and start choosing yourself as the most magnetic woman in the room, in his memory, and in his body.

This isn't about chasing him. It's about becoming the only thing that feels *real* when everything else fades. You're not a ghost or a thought. You're a pulse. A craving. A fire. A frequency his nervous system can't forget. And once you've rewired that craving into his core—emotionally, sensually, energetically—he'll spend the rest of his life trying to feel that alive again.

Chapter 7: BURNING DESIRE

The Step-by-Step Ritual That Makes Him Burn for You

There comes a moment when a woman stops waiting for something to happen—and begins *willing* it into motion. Not through force. Not through performance. But through the focused transmission of her own energy—calm, clear, and deeply charged.

This is that moment for you.

Because what you're about to learn isn't just another visualization. It's not a seduction script or a spiritual metaphor wrapped in soft language. This is real. This is about *impact*—emotional, physical, energetic. The kind of impact that lands in a man's body before he has time to rationalize it. The kind that makes his skin prickle, his stomach twist, his heart race—for reasons he can't explain.

Remote seduction doesn't rely on proximity. It's not about looks, words, or even whether he still thinks he wants you. Because once you know how to speak to his nervous system directly—none of that matters.

What matters is what his body remembers.

What matters is the signal you send.

What matters is how vividly you imprint the experience—so that it becomes something he feels, not something he thinks.

This technique is about more than arousal. It's about emotional authority. It's about tapping into the deepest craving centers of his mind and leaving an energetic residue that lingers, even after the moment has passed. He may brush it off. He may distract himself. But his body will remember. And the memory will have *you* in it.

You don't need to understand every mechanism for this to work. But if you want to influence a man at this level, you do need to understand one thing:

The brain cannot distinguish between imagination and reality when intense emotion is present.

Let that sink in.

To your nervous system—and his—*what is vividly imagined, especially when combined with physical sensation and emotion, gets stored as memory.*

This is the science behind remote seduction. You're not "pretending" something into being. You are rehearsing an experience so vividly, with so much sensory detail and emotional charge, that it leaves a physical impression on your body and a psychic imprint on his. Whether he's asleep, distracted, or dating someone new, he will feel it.

And when done correctly, this ritual doesn't just seduce him.

It *rewires* him.

Let's begin.

→Step 1: Relax the Body to Activate the Channel

Your body is the antenna.

Before you can transmit energy, influence, or emotion—you must first shift your own nervous system into a receptive, open state. Not the high-alert tension most of us live in, and not the artificial calm of distraction. This requires a deliberate downshift. A full surrender.

Start by lying flat on your back. Choose a space where you feel supported—your bed, the couch, even the floor is fine. What matters is stillness. Comfort. Privacy. No music, no background noise, no visual clutter.

Uncross your arms and legs so energy flows smoothly and evenly. Let your hands rest palms-up beside your hips. Let your breath move gently in and out without controlling it. Then begin to notice the surface beneath you. Feel the weight of your body pressing down—your shoulder blades, hips, heels. Let gravity do the work.

This is not just relaxation. This is the preparation for energetic influence.

Now close your eyes and begin the 4-7-8 breath:

→ Inhale gently for a count of 4

→ Hold your breath for a count of 7

→ Exhale slowly and fully for a count of 8

Repeat this cycle three or four times. You don't need to force anything. Just stay present with the rhythm. As you breathe, your brain begins to shift out of beta (the alert, analyzing state) and into alpha—the dreamy, magnetic state of imagination and subconscious access.

Alpha brainwaves are where you become most suggestible—and most powerful.

This is the gateway.

As you breathe and soften, you'll begin to feel a sense of expansion. Like your awareness is stretching beyond your skin. You may feel warm, floaty, slightly buzzed. That's good. That's your nervous system shifting from doing to *receiving.*

This state matters because energy moves most easily when resistance is low. In a tense, thinking state, you're sending mixed signals. But in alpha, your energy becomes coherent—smooth, directed, magnetic.

And here's what most women never realize: when you're in this state and you tune into his energy, *he* can feel it. Even if he doesn't know why. Your energy field becomes larger, more radiant, more noticeable. Like a ripple in the air around him, his body will register something.

He might get a sudden chill.

He might feel distracted or aroused.

He might remember you out of nowhere and not know why.

This is your signal arriving.

Once you feel yourself relax into this open, dreamy state—stay there. No effort. No performance. Just breath, softness, and a quiet sense of inner power.

You are now the transmitter.

You are the source.

And he's already starting to tune in.

➜ Step 2: See Him Across the Space

With your body relaxed and your energy open, bring him into focus.

In your mind's eye, see yourself standing in a quiet, empty space. Somewhere wide and open—an empty street at dusk or a parking lot washed in silver moonlight. It's not dark, but it's hushed. Like the world is paused. Like something important is about to happen.

This space belongs to you.

Now look out across the distance—30 or 40 feet away—and there he is.

Not a symbol. Not a shape. *Him.*

You don't have to force the image. Let your energy shape it

➜ What is he wearing?

➜ How is he standing?

➜ Is he walking slowly, aimlessly, or simply existing in the space like he doesn't know why he's there?

➜ What's the texture of the air—warm, charged, still?

You're not looking at him passively. You're preparing to send something into his space—into his field.

Now breathe in.

And from the center of your being, with total emotional clarity, send the command:

"Michael!"

"Michael, look at me!"

Not a whisper. A *blast*.

You shout it in your mind with such sharp emotional intensity that it travels straight through the invisible space between you like a spear made of sound and memory.

And in that instant—you *hit him*.

You don't see it on the surface. But you feel it in his field.

His energy ripples—subtly but undeniably. Like the echo of a bell that's just been struck. His awareness shifts. His attention stumbles.

It's not a conscious thought like *"Did someone call my name?"* It's a *recognition*.

A jolt in his subconscious.

A flare of emotional electricity.

A feeling that someone just stepped into his field.

This is the moment where you pierce his energetic bubble—the invisible shield most people walk around with, protecting their inner world. Your energy just breached that barrier, not with words, but with emotion. And even if he doesn't understand what happened, *he feels it.*

There's an internal interruption.

His mental focus fragments.

His field stirs.

He might blink. He might shift his weight. His eyes may search the space like he's looking for something he can't name. This is not fantasy. This is real. His subconscious just received your signal—and it's trying to make sense of the intrusion.

And then… he sees you.

You feel the snap of recognition. A sharp psychic click, like a lock turning. Something in him anchors to you. His energy stops moving outward—and starts moving toward you.

He begins to walk. Deliberately. Like the air just changed. Like he knows, on some deep level, that *you* are the one who pulled him here.

And as he moves closer, something begins to open in him.

He doesn't understand it. But the emotional climate inside him has shifted.

The connection has been made.

And now his field is adjusting—registering you as something it's supposed to track, respond to, and remember.

You're not just imagining a scene.

You're *entering his space.*

You're not controlling him. You're not manipulating.

You're simply becoming unavoidable.

→ Step 3: Connect to Him

He's standing just a few feet away now.

You can feel his presence in your field—thick, charged, undeniable. He's not just in your mind anymore. He's *here*. Close enough to touch. Close enough to feel the atmosphere shift between your bodies.

Your eyes meet.

Not in fantasy—but in focus. In connection.

You don't need to see every detail of his body anymore. You're locked into the most potent part of him—his gaze. His awareness. His emotional center. You're not just looking at his face. You're *inside* the experience of being this close to him— breathing the same energy, standing in shared space.

Hold that eye contact.

Even if it's imagined—your nervous system can't tell the difference. Neither can his.

Because right now, something deeper than logic is happening.

There's a stillness in the space around you. A magnetic tension, like something ancient just clicked into place. It feels like déjà vu, but heavier. *Familiar, but new.* The air between you feels thick with possibility.

Now let your own energy soften.

You're not pushing. You're not reaching. You're simply opening—emotionally, energetically. Let yourself radiate what you feel: love, hunger, vulnerability, confidence.

That emotion isn't just yours—it becomes the medium through which connection deepens.

And now, call his name—silently, powerfully. Three times.

"Michael…"

"Michael…"

"Michael…"

Let each repetition be slower, deeper, more emotionally charged than the last. Like a beacon sent across a vast sea—your voice calling him home.

As you speak his name, feel the shift.

Suddenly, the space between you tightens. You can almost hear the psychic click as the connection locks in.

Now imagine a brilliant silver thread—pure, electric—shooting from the center of your forehead (your third eye) straight into his. Not a flimsy line. A living pulse. Thick with energy. Hot with clarity.

It doesn't float or drift. It *snaps* into place.

Like it was always there, waiting to be activated.

And the moment it does, his system registers it.

It's not conscious. He doesn't "realize" anything.

But something deep inside him—beneath thought—feels claimed.

Like he's just been seen… touched… remembered in a way no one else ever has.

This is what happens when you project energy through the third eye:

His mirror neurons begin firing as if you're physically near

His limbic brain starts translating your emotional tone into sensation

His subconscious flags you as important—*crucial*, even—without knowing why

He may feel dizzy. Focused. Lit up. Haunted.

And now—send the words.

Not out loud. Not with force. With emotion.

"You missed me."

"You desire me."

"You want me and only me."

Let each phrase ride the cord like a current of electricity, dripping straight into his subconscious. These aren't affirmations. They're *imprints*—emotional data his body begins absorbing as if they're his own inner knowing.

He doesn't "hear" them the way he hears a voice.

He *feels* them—like inner truth rising from a forgotten part of him.

Something stirs in his field. A restlessness. A searching. A craving without a label.

Because your energy is now inside him.

And the connection can't be undone.

→ Step 4: Touch Him. Seduce Him. Own Him.

He's here now—fully inside your field, tethered to you by the silver thread of emotional connection. You're no longer just imagining him. You're engaging him.

He may be far away in the physical world. But his energetic body is standing right in front of you—open, sensitive, responsive. And your energy has become the force shaping his experience.

This moment can—and should—become sexual.

Because sexual energy is more than arousal. It's memory. Power. Magnetism. It's the deepest imprint the body can hold.

If you've already been intimate with him, let yourself *go back.*

Choose a moment when you were completely connected. When time disappeared. When it felt like there was no separation between your body and his. Don't just remember it. **Relive it.**

Drop into that memory as if it's *happening now.* Feel his weight. His heat. The rhythm of your breath against his. The way your body opened for him—not just physically, but emotionally. The way your hearts beat together when everything else went still.

Let it flood you.

Let your body respond.

Because your body's reaction is part of the signal. And every flicker of heat, every wave of pleasure, every breathless moment you recreate—*he feels it*. Not logically. Not like a thought. But as a disruption in his energy field. A spike of desire. A shift in focus. A memory he didn't know was still alive.

And if you've never had sex with him?

Create it.

In your mind's eye, imagine him as clearly as possible—his scent, the way his skin would feel under your hands, the tension in his jaw, the look in his eyes just before he gives in.

Then imagine what you would do.

Not as a performance. Not as a fantasy to impress him. But as a real experience, grounded in your own desire. Let your imagination become the stage for a full-body emotional encounter.

Let it build.

Let yourself *want* him.

Let your mind guide you into the feeling of skin on skin... lips on neck... breath against collarbone. Imagine the heat rising between you as clothes fall away. The sound of your voice in his ear. The tension. The hunger. The surrender.

Don't rush it. Let it rise like a storm.

Feel his body responding to yours.

Feel his hips moving with you.

Feel the emotion—yes, emotion—behind the intensity.

Because the truth is, when sex is laced with emotion, it becomes **unforgettable.** That's when it imprints. That's when it becomes more than pleasure—it becomes a *need*.

Your body may begin to tremble.

Your breath may quicken.

You might even reach orgasm in real time.

Let it happen.

That release sends a pulse through the energetic cord—like a detonation of desire. He may not know what it was. But somewhere in his field, he *feels* it.

A ripple of electricity.

A tightening in his chest.

A moment of arousal that comes out of nowhere.

And here's the part most women don't expect:

Sometimes, he'll feel it *in real time.*

He might get flushed or lightheaded out of nowhere. He might feel turned on in the middle of the day and not know why. He might even wake from a dream—sweaty, hard, confused—with *you* in his mind.

That's not a coincidence.

That's your energy.

You've entered his subconscious and triggered a physical response—one he can't trace, but one his body *remembers*.

And once your energy has entered him that deeply—he will never fully forget it.

You've now planted not just a scene, but a **somatic memory**—the kind the body holds even when the mind tries to move on. Every time he sees you, dreams of you, hears your name, or even touches someone else… part of him will remember.

Because this wasn't just imagined.

It was *transmitted.*

And energy doesn't lie.

You've touched him.

Claimed him.

And carved your name into the deepest emotional layer of his desire.

And you did it with nothing but energy, intention, and presence.

This is where remote seduction becomes *real.*

And it's only just begun.

→ Step 5: Let Him Touch You

Now that the energy is moving between you—thick, alive, undeniable—let him reach for you.

Not with logic. Not with words. With instinct.

Allow his energy to move toward yours—not because you're pulling, but because you've become impossible to resist. Your field is magnetic now. It's glowing with memory, emotion, heat. And his system, consciously or not, begins to lean in.

Let it unfold without force.

He steps closer—not physically, but psychically. The bond between you tightens. And his energetic body begins to mirror yours. His presence becomes more focused, more charged. It's as if his subconscious has received the signal and is now sending one back—unspoken but deeply felt.

You feel him reach for you—not just with hands, but with energy.

His field wraps around yours like a second skin. Protective. Possessive. Familiar.

You might imagine his arms around your waist… his chest against yours… your head tucked into the warmth of his neck. But this isn't just about fantasy imagery. It's about what it feels like to be wanted that deeply. To be held energetically. To be felt.

His embrace becomes emotional—not just physical.

It carries the weight of everything unspoken.

The longing.

The regret.

The hunger.

The tenderness that breaks open just beneath the desire.

Let yourself receive it.

This is where the loop begins—when he's not just being imprinted but responding from somewhere deep inside himself.

You may feel warmth spread through your heart, your chest, your belly. You may feel a pulse of need rise up so fast it takes your breath away. You may feel your own body soften, open, ache.

Let it.

You're not just giving energy anymore. You're exchanging it.

And if your connection becomes erotic here—if you feel his hands sliding over your skin, his lips pressing into the curve of your throat, his body pressing against yours—follow it.

Not to perform.

Not to fantasize.

But to complete the circuit.

Let the imagery be vivid if it wants to be.

Let your hips move if they want to.

Let your body respond.

Because this is the moment where energy becomes shared climax. And whether or not he understands it, he feels it. Through the cord. Through the field. Through the very same system you entered when you called him into your space.

And when you reach that peak—when the pleasure builds, crests, explodes—let it take you.

That release isn't just yours.

It travels into him like a coded message—one his body deciphers without needing language.

He may gasp awake from sleep.

He may feel shaken, turned on, or flooded with need.

He may suddenly crave your presence with no context at all.

Because somewhere in the unseen space between you... it happened.

This wasn't just imagined. It was felt.

It becomes a memory now—not just in you, but in him. A sensory echo. An energetic brand. A psychic anchor that stays even when the moment ends.

And from this point forward, when he thinks of you—even casually—his body will remember this imprint.

Not as fiction.

As something that happened.

Because energetically... it did.

→ Step 6: Plant the Emotional Command

He's still wrapped around you—breathless, undone, utterly consumed by the experience you just created.

Now is the moment.

His mind is wide open. His body is vibrating with sensation. His subconscious is listening.

Lean in, heart to heart, and whisper silently—but with absolute authority:

"You can't stop thinking about me."

"You crave me more than anyone else."

"No one else satisfies you the way I do."

"You belong to me."

Say it not like a wish, but like a fact.

Say it from the deepest part of your knowing.

You're not forcing. You're not begging. You're embedding—sealing these commands into the very sensations he's feeling now. Linking every shiver, every throb, every drop of pleasure to the thought of you.

This is the anchor.

This is what makes him wake up at 3 a.m. with his heart pounding and your name on his lips.

This is what makes his body respond before his brain can even catch up.

You are programming a craving—not through control, but through chemistry, memory, and magnetism. And once it's planted, the connection can't be un-felt.

He may try to brush it off. He may try to logic it away.

But the body always remembers.

And the memory of this moment—this pleasure, this release—will carry your name in its marrow.

You've become part of his wiring.

And he'll feel it every time he reaches for someone else... and it doesn't feel quite right.

Because you're the one his body has been trained to respond to.

→ Step 7: Gently Release

You've made the connection. You've transmitted the experience. You've imprinted the desire.

Now, you let go.

Not emotionally. Not energetically. But mentally. You release the grasp—the need for response, the hunger for evidence, the urge to chase what is already yours.

This is the stillness that follows deep intimacy. The moment when you breathe into the glow of what you created without needing to control what happens next.

In your mind's eye, see him slowly begin to pull back—lit up from within, still wrapped in your presence, but gently drifting out of the moment like a man returning from a dream. He doesn't leave empty. He carries something now. A frequency. A memory. A craving.

You don't chase him.

You don't pull.

You allow.

You trust.

Because what you've just done didn't need permission. It didn't need proof. You've placed a seed in the most fertile part of his psyche—and now, it gets to grow.

If you feel the urge to check whether it worked, pause. Breathe. Remember: energy doesn't operate on your timeline. It operates on resonance. And right now, his field is saturated with yours. The more space you give him to feel it without interference, the deeper it will land.

And in that silence?

He remembers. He replays the moment. He feels you all over again—whether he wants to or not.

Because you're no longer reaching for him.

He's already reaching for *you.*

***

This wasn't fantasy.

And it wasn't fiction.

This was energetic reality.

What you just did wasn't a daydream. It was a deliberate act of influence—a conscious creation, encoded with desire and sent straight into his subconscious.

You didn't seduce him with your body. You seduced him with your soul.

And that is power.

Not the kind that manipulates.

The kind that awakens.

This technique is not about obsession or control. It's about reclaiming your energy and directing it with precision, emotion, and confidence. It's about making him feel you long after you've gone silent. It's about taking up space in his system not by force, but by frequency.

And once you've done it well, there's no mistaking it.

Because the craving becomes real. The emotional echo becomes constant. And you—without even touching him—become unforgettable.

A friend of mine once confessed something that stayed with me. She had been experimenting with the technique but wasn't sure if it was real. "It felt so vivid—so sensual and intense," she told me. "But then I wondered if I'd just let my imagination run wild. Like... did anything actually happen?" She wanted to know. Not just believe—but know.

So she tested it on someone who once meant everything to her. Her ex. A man she had broken up with after discovering he'd been secretly online dating behind her back. The betrayal was brutal. She hadn't just lost trust—she had lost her sense of safety. They hadn't spoken since the breakup. But one part of her still wanted him to feel it. To remember what they had. Not through words. Not through confrontation. But through energy. She didn't want closure. She wanted impact.

She used the technique on him. She visualized, connected, and poured all the love, longing, and sensual intensity of their time together back into his subconscious. She didn't tell me how many times. I didn't ask. But then... something shifted and she felt it immediately. He came back. Not casually. Not calmly. Desperately. Obsessively.

Within weeks he was texting, calling, leaving emotional voicemails late at night. He even reached out to their mutual friend and confided his desperation. "I don't know what you did to me," he told her more than once. "I couldn't stop thinking about you." The irony? She didn't want him anymore. By the time he showed up, begging for a second chance, she had cut the cord. Emotionally. Energetically. She no longer needed his validation—because the power had come back to her.

But he didn't give up. It took him six long months of consistent effort—changing, growing, proving himself—before she agreed to see him again. And a few months ago, they got married. She told me it was never about getting him back. It was about taking back her power and making him feel it. And that once she did, he was the one who couldn't walk away. Because the energy had spoken louder than words ever could.

You're not here to play small. You're here to master the power of your own energy, your own body, your own influence. And this technique—when practiced with confidence and intention—makes you unforgettable. You don't have to seduce with your body. You can seduce with your soul. And when you do it well, he won't know what hit him. But you will. Because you created it. And you're just getting started.

Chapter 8: Orgasmic Energy

Send Pleasure Without Touch—And Make Him Feel It

What if you don't have a man in your life right now? Simple. Go get one.

You don't have to flash your cleavage. You don't have to giggle over a cocktail. You don't even have to move from your barstool. You can have a man across the room—across the street—across the city—begin to burn for you just by using your mind.

This technique is fun, magnetic, and almost too easy once you get the hang of it. And he'll never even know what hit him.

It starts like this:

➔ Look around the room.

➔ Find someone who catches your eye—even slightly.

➔ Just notice a few details.

Maybe it's the way his jacket fits across his shoulders. Maybe it's the way his mouth curves when he smiles. You don't need to memorize him. You just need enough to summon his image when you look away. That's it.

The moment you notice him—and he notices you—you are already energetically linked. You're entangled. The game is on.

Now, without staring at him, without being obvious:

➔ Close your eyes briefly or glance down at your phone.

➔ In your mind, yell out to him: "Hey, you. You feel me. You want me."

Imagine it loud. Commanding. Magnetic.

You may even visualize yourself brushing past him... breathing softly into his ear... pressing your lips lightly against his neck. No names necessary. Your energy knows where to go.

If you want, you can simply "breathe" into his ear mentally. Soft, warm, inviting. That alone will make some men turn around and look at you—sensing the charge without understanding why.

If you're feeling bolder—and you're talking to a man casually:

➔ Visualize running your fingers down his forearm as you chat.

➔ Or brushing your hand along his chest.

➔ Or tracing the back of his neck with featherlight fingertips.

You can do this invisibly, while smiling politely, sipping your drink, making small talk. And if your energy is strong enough, he will start reacting physically. Shifting in his chair. Flushing. Fidgeting. Feeling the tension build without a clue where it's coming from.

Want to light up a man who's just an acquaintance? Someone who never paid you much attention before? Visualize it.

➔ See yourself giving him the kind of sexual experience that makes his soul leave his body.

➔ Feel every touch. Every kiss. Every moan.

➔ Make it so vivid you could almost swear it happened.

Then watch what happens the next time he sees you. He won't know why, but he'll look at you differently. Longer. Hungrier. You've already woven yourself into his energy field.

One of my favorite success stories came from a client who had broken up with a man she no longer wanted. For fun—and maybe just a little revenge—she decided to keep sending him these energy charges once a week. Five minutes. That's all.

She would spend five minutes flooding him with memories of touch, breath, skin, heat. And even though they hadn't been together for over a year, he couldn't get over her. He dated other women, but none could hold his attention. He'd text her late at night. He'd "accidentally" run into her places. He confessed he felt a constant craving for her he couldn't explain.

He thought he was losing his mind. He wasn't. He was just receiving exactly what she was sending.

→ As you visualize the scene—his breath, his touch, his hunger—let yourself respond physically. Not performatively. Just naturally.

→ Let your hand brush your collarbone, your thigh, your neck—anywhere you want him to feel it.

This isn't just for you. It's for the link. Your body is the transmitter. The more real it feels to you, the more real it becomes for him.

Studies on remote intention and biofield awareness have shown that the human body can respond to emotional stimuli—

even from a distance—when the sender is focused and emotionally charged. Translation? Your energy is not just a vibe. It's a signal his nervous system can pick up—even if he doesn't know why.

If you want to practice this technique without risking your target, you can even try it with a willing friend.

➜ Agree to a simple experiment: You'll send her a mental "hello" at a specific time. She'll write down anything she feels, hears, or senses.

You don't even have to make it sexual (unless you both agree). The point is to prove to yourself how easily your energy reaches someone else—especially when they're open and expecting it.

Just remember: Energy is sticky. Once you impress an idea onto someone's subconscious, it's very hard for them to un-feel it. Even if they can't logically explain why.

A quick personal example: After a breakup, I once tried reconnecting with a man who had completely shut down emotionally. He wasn't just angry—he had built walls around himself. Concrete. Steel. Solid.

When I first tried sending energy his way, it felt like throwing a paper airplane at a fortress. But I didn't give up. Instead of pushing, I softened. I flooded him with love, forgiveness, longing. And waited.

Days passed. Weeks passed. Then one day, out of nowhere, he called me. He was sobbing. Saying he missed me so much it hurt. That he didn't understand it. That it hit him like a freight train.

The truth? It wasn't sudden. It was the buildup of all the emotions I had been sending through the walls—waiting for the moment his defenses cracked. Energy always finds a way.

And if you're wondering, "Can this really work for me, even if I've never had sex? Never kissed a man? Never even seen a penis in person?"—the answer is yes.

I've had women write to me—women who had never been touched, never been kissed, and didn't know what physical intimacy felt like—asking if this would still work. After talking with them and guiding them through it, the results were undeniable.

Not only did it work—it worked beautifully. In fact, the build-up, the energy, the sensual charge they created in their minds often made the eventual connection even more intense and emotionally unforgettable.

Sometimes, sex is better in the mind than in real life—but when you use remote seduction, you're blending the two. You're creating a real, energetic encounter that enhances both fantasy and reality.

Final note: You can do this anywhere, anytime.

→ In line at the grocery store.

→ Sitting at a red light.

→ Curling up in bed.

You don't need candles, rituals, or ceremonies. You just need focus. Emotion. And a willingness to let yourself truly feel the experience you're creating.

Because when you do? He will, too.

And nothing—not time, not distance, not even logic—will stop the fire you lit inside him.

Burn, baby, burn.

Chapter 9: Master-Level Remote Seduction Techniques

Advanced Psychic Linking, Soul Bonding & Energy Merging

Some of the best moments in life are the ones you can't tell anyone about. And Remote Seduction creates more of those moments than anything else I've ever taught.

Before we dive deeper, let me give you a little word of advice: Just because you can step into someone else's energy field doesn't always mean you should. Yes—it's possible to energetically project yourself right into another person's body. Yes—you can feel their emotions, their desires, their attraction for you in a way that's shockingly real.

But remember—when you entangle yourself that deeply, you're not just connecting to the parts of them you want. You're touching everything: their dreams, their fears, their hidden emotional baggage. If you're sensitive (and you will become more sensitive the deeper you go), you may pick up on energy you didn't bargain for.

Still, for the adventurous spirits among you, here's the technique:

➔ **First**, relax your body completely. Use 4-7-8 breathing if you like: Inhale for 4 counts. Hold for 7 counts. Exhale for 8 counts. Tell yourself mentally: "Sleepy, sleepy, sleepy..." until your mind drifts inward. You're aiming for the Alpha state—where brainwaves slow, reality blurs, and your subconscious opens.

→ **Second**, create a vivid 3D image of the person you desire. Feel them standing in front of you. See them clearly—the way their clothes drape their body, the glint in their eyes, the heat radiating from their skin.

→ **Third**, imagine yourself stepping gently out of your own body—like a spirit made of golden light. You walk toward him and slip inside his energetic form, like sliding your hands into a pair of gloves. This is called energetic merging—overlaying your consciousness onto his subtle body.

You are not forcing. You are aligning. You are inhabiting the vibration of his being—and because intention rules energy, he feels it instantly on a subconscious level.

→ **Fourth**, feel what he feels. Let yourself absorb his desire, his hunger, his ache for you. You're no longer "imagining" connection. You are the connection. You are inside his emotional field, amplifying and awakening everything you want him to feel.

→ **Fifth**, while you are inside him, gently plant the thoughts you want him to think: "I can't stop thinking about her..." "She's irresistible..." "No other woman could ever satisfy me..." "I have to have her." Let these thoughts ripple outward through his mind like ink spreading through water. The more vividly you experience them, the more deeply they will root inside him.

→ **Sixth**, as the emotions and arousal build, imagine two cords forming: One from your solar plexus (your power center) to his. One from your sacral/sexual center to his. If it feels natural, add a laser beam of golden light from your third eye directly into his. These connections aren't just fantasy. In energy work—and in quantum theory—they are real transmission lines of information and emotion. You are building a bridge between your subconscious and his.

→ **Seventh**, when the emotional and energetic bond feels complete, gently step back out of his body. Return to your own beautiful energy field. Take a deep breath and feel yourself fully back inside yourself—strong, radiant, sovereign.

Important: After merging, always visualize both yourself and him surrounded in golden light. You can even imagine mirrored spheres reflecting outward—to ensure that no energetic debris, no emotional fragments, stay attached. You want clean, pure, vibrant energy between you—not lingering entanglement unless you choose it. Energetic hygiene is sacred when you are playing at this level.

A few things to know about energetic merging: When you step inside him, you will experience a new level of intimacy—a depth that physical touch alone cannot create. This is why he will feel so magnetically drawn to you afterward without knowing why. You're not just sending desire. You're weaving your presence into the very fabric of his being.

This level of merging is more than fantasy. It's energetic imprinting. When you allow yourself to feel what he feels—to see through his eyes, crave through his skin, ache through his body—

you aren't just seducing him... You're becoming part of his emotional memory.

Later, he won't be able to explain why certain images, thoughts, or feelings stir him unexpectedly. But you'll know. You planted them. And now, they live inside him like a flame waiting for your spark.

This technique works in a way that echoes the quantum concept of entanglement—where two particles, once connected, continue to influence each other across time and space. Similarly, when you link your energy to his at this level, you are embedding emotional and energetic data into his subconscious in a way that bypasses logic.

Heart-based studies have shown that our electromagnetic fields extend far beyond the body—and that emotional information is transmitted through those fields whether we're conscious of it or not. This isn't science fiction. It's subtle, measurable, and increasingly supported by research on human biofields and nonlocal consciousness.

You are not working at the level of logic, resistance, or social masks. You are connecting at the soul, energy, and feeling level—the place where real attraction, obsession, and emotional attachment are born.

By now, you've practiced the spark of fantasy, the pull of craving, the imprint of desire. But merging? This is where all of it converges. This is where seduction stops being about persuasion—and starts becoming memory.

I've had clients who had never experienced sex, who had never even kissed a man, ask me if this could work for them. The answer is not only yes—it often works even better. Because when you have no physical memories to pull from, your mind weaves desire in its purest, most vivid form—uncontaminated by past disappointments.

Remote Seduction lets you create passion so real, so overwhelming, that it can eclipse even physical reality.

I've had women tell me their POIs reached out in shock, asking, "Were you thinking about me? I swear I could feel you last night." I've had women, after months or years of distance, reignite lost loves and attract entirely new ones—without lifting a finger. Not because they "tried harder." But because they merged deeper. Because they learned to seduce with energy, not effort. And you can too.

➜ **Try This**: Before sleep tonight, choose someone you feel drawn to. Relax. Breathe. Visualize yourself stepping into his energetic body—not to chase or beg—but to show him what it feels like to be loved, desired, and possessed by you. Plant a thought. Feel the craving. Then slowly step back into your own energy field and fall asleep.

This is only the beginning.

Chapter 10 – The Magnetic Power of a Text Message

How to Penetrate His Mind, Trigger His Body, and Anchor Yourself With Just a Few Words

What if I told you a single text could make him hard, haunted, or emotionally hooked for days?

It's not wishful thinking. It's biology, psychology, and energy—wrapped in the innocent ping of a screen.

Text messages aren't just words. They're subconscious anchors. They bypass logic, land straight in his nervous system, and loop in his brain long after you've hit send. Especially when you send them right after Remote Seduction—when his field is already cracked open and craving you.

The truth? This is one of the most overlooked tools in remote seduction. And in my other book—*Texting & Sexting*—we go even deeper. I teach you how to combine sexual energy, emotional imprinting, and exact word structures to get under his skin and stay there. But here's the short version.

Words That Penetrate:

Text messages bypass layers of resistance. They land directly in his hand, often while he's alone, relaxed, or caught off guard. No makeup. No voice. No social filter. Just pure words and emotional imprint.

Studies show that reading an emotionally charged message lights up the same brain centers as hearing a lover's voice. It creates a felt sense—his heart rate may spike, his pupils may dilate, and yes, his body can physically respond.

In a 2022 neurobiology study, subjects who received flirtatious or emotionally weighted texts showed measurable changes in oxytocin and cortisol—the love and stress hormones. In other words, a well-timed text can seduce or destabilize his nervous system. You're not just sending a message. You're triggering chemistry.

Why a Text Lingers Longer Than a Touch:

Texting is asynchronous seduction. That means he can reread your words. Revisit the moment. Loop your tone, your timing, the hidden meanings. A well-crafted text message creates reverberation. He'll check it twice. Three times. Screenshot it. Think about it later in the shower. Think about it again when he's bored. And again at midnight.

It doesn't fade—it burns in.

This is why ghost texts—messages with emotional hooks and no follow-up—drive men insane. They build tension with no release. It's digital foreplay.

Energetic Transfer Through Text:

Sounds woo-woo, right? But here's the thing: intention carries energy, no matter the medium. Think about it—have you ever felt the vibe in a text message? You knew when someone was angry, cold, horny, or obsessed—even if the words were neutral.

That's not magic. That's frequency transfer. You send your energy with your words.

And when you combine sexual energy with emotionally loaded language, the impact is atomic.

In fact, your energetic intention can prime a text before you hit send. Want to try it?

Close your eyes and feel what you want him to feel: longing, arousal, curiosity.

Imagine your fingertips glowing with heat and electricity.

Now write the message.

Just before hitting send, whisper his name in your mind and beam the message like a bullet of desire straight to his chest.

You've just weaponized your words.

When to Send (and When Not To)

Texting after sex? Too soon.

Texting at 11:11 PM after disappearing all day? That's a spell.

Texting during a high-energy moment, when he's with friends or working?

Missed.

Texting during his downtime, when he's craving stimulation, sex, or connection? Bullseye.

Texting isn't just about what you say. It's about when and how he receives it.

Real-Life Story: A Cold Relationship Reignited by Remote Seduction Text

One of my readers had been in a long-term relationship for years, but the spark was long gone. Her partner was sweet—but intimacy had become mechanical, rare, or nonexistent. She felt invisible. I suggested she try the remote seduction technique we've already covered—along with one new element: *texting*.

She didn't send anything explicit at first. Just energy. Then one night, after doing the exercise, she wrote:

"Don't ask me why, but I can still feel your breath on my neck from that night."

He texted back instantly:

"Are you trying to kill me? I've been thinking about that all day."

That night, he initiated the most passionate sex they'd had in years.

She began sending him subtle, emotionally charged texts only after doing the technique—when the energy was fresh. Each time, he responded with more intensity. Within two weeks, they were having sex again. And more than that, they were laughing, touching, connecting. Like it was new.

What to Send

This isn't about copy-paste messages. It's about opening loops in his mind that only you can close.

Try these examples as a jumping-off point:

- "Thinking about that thing you said…"
- "You'd laugh if you knew what I'm thinking right now."
- "Not sure what's gotten into me lately. I blame you."
- "I keep replaying that night."
- "You make it hard to concentrate sometimes."

For existing relationships that have gone cold, try one of these:

- "I had a dream about you last night. Should I be concerned?"
- "I miss the way your voice sounded when you couldn't catch your breath."
- "Do you ever think about how good it used to be?"
- "We used to be dangerous together. Kind of miss that."
- "If you could read my mind right now, you'd probably blush."

Each one is a spark. What he does with it is up to him—but his body will respond whether he wants it to or not.

Bold Erotic Texts to Reignite Desire

These are perfect for long-term relationships that need heat, or for women who feel unseen and want to shift the dynamic without begging for attention. These aren't texts that ask for love—they command attention and stir desire from the inside out.

- "I don't want to talk. I want your hands on me, your mouth on mine, and your body making me forget everything else."

- "I just remembered that thing you did with your tongue… and now I can't stop squirming."
- "You know what I miss? The way you used to pin me down like you couldn't get close enough."
- "If I whispered everything I want you to do to me right now… we wouldn't make it past the front door."
- "I had a dream last night. You were behind me, breathing in my ear, and I woke up wet. You should've been there."
- "What would you do if I showed up right now wearing nothing but a smile and my perfume?"
- "Tonight, I don't want soft. I want the version of you that makes me ache all day after."
- "I've been good all week. Don't you think it's time you ruined my innocence again?"

These texts work best when sent with confidence—not insecurity. They're not about fishing for compliments or asking to be wanted. They're a reminder of what you awaken in him when you stop holding back your sensual power.

If You're in a Relationship That's Gone Cold

Try these more emotionally evocative lines to reignite the spark. They work by activating his emotional memory and inviting connection, not confrontation.

- "I miss the way you used to look at me… like I was the only thing you saw."

- "Do you ever think about the way it felt in the beginning—before life got in the way?"
- "I don't need a fancy dinner. I just want the man who used to pull me close without asking."
- "Sometimes I replay that night we couldn't keep our hands off each other. Do you ever think about it too?"
- "I know life gets busy... but I miss being your favorite distraction."

These are quiet invitations. They don't blame. They don't beg. They whisper to the part of him that *remembers...* and that's where the desire lives.

A Final Note

You don't need to be a writer or a seductress to send a powerful text. You just need to feel something—and send it with intention. Because what you're really doing isn't texting.

You're programming.

You're seducing his subconscious.

You're anchoring yourself into his emotional body.

And that's the kind of message he'll never forget.

Why This Belongs in Remote Seduction

Because this *is* remote seduction.

You're reaching into his mind with zero physical effort. You're guiding emotion, energy, and memory. And if you've done the earlier techniques—entanglement, projection, erotic imprinting—your text won't just make him react...

...it'll make him spiral.

He'll associate you with pleasure. He'll crave your energy. And he'll start chasing the high you created—even if he doesn't know how you did it.

Because once your words enter his nervous system, they're not just messages.

They're anchors.

They're spells.

They're energy he can't shake.

And that's exactly the point.

Chapter 11: What If He Doesn't Respond?

Real Stories, Deep Energy, and Why He Still Feels You

Let's talk about something nobody warns you about: Sometimes, even when you're doing everything right—Even when your energy is hot, pure, and focused:

You might not see immediate proof.

You might be thinking, "Is this working? Is he even feeling it?"

Let me tell you a story.

When I first began experimenting with these techniques—way before I ever published a word about them—I had an ex we'll call John.

Handsome.

Wealthy.

Intelligent.

He could have had any woman he wanted. And trust me, they were lined up.

But after I broke up with him—and after I used the PW technique and this Remote Seduction method—you know what happened?

He couldn't move on.

For years.

He hired private detectives to follow me.

He rented cars so I wouldn't recognize him—and parked three doors down, hiding in the bushes, just to watch me.

He even slept in rental cars, parked right in front of my house overnight. He was still asking bartenders about me at our favorite restaurant seven years later.

Seven. Years.

And no, he never married.

Never got into a long-term relationship again. Despite everything he had to offer—and everything the world offered him back—he was still entangled with me.

That's the power of these techniques. That's the power of real energetic connection.

Once you penetrate a man's subconscious mind this way— once you wire desire, longing, and emotional hunger into his system—it doesn't just evaporate. It lasts.

Think of it like the Energizer Bunny of emotional attachment: It keeps going... and going... and going.

That's why I always tell my readers: Be careful what you ask for.

Because when you do this technique with real passion, real connection, and real feeling—it becomes real inside him too.

Even if he fights it.

Even if life pulls him in other directions.

You'll still live in a part of his mind he can't erase.

Reader Success Stories: He Felt It. They Always Do.

This method isn't just a theory. It's been tested, used, and trusted by women from every walk of life—some spiritual, some skeptical, some who had never even kissed the man they were attracting.

One woman had been blocked by her ex for over six months. No contact. No updates. Nothing. She used the technique nightly for just two weeks—soft music, candlelight, and pure intention. He unblocked her out of nowhere and texted, *"I had the weirdest dream about you. You felt so real... like I woke up missing you."*

Another woman used this on a man she'd never met in person—just a voice on the phone. She described him as powerful, masculine, emotionally unavailable. After three remote sessions, he called her with his voice shaking.

"I don't know what you did to me... but I've been hard since Tuesday."

Then there was the woman in a cold marriage. They hadn't touched each other in months. One night she lit a candle, tapped into the memory of their first kiss, and sent it to him energetically. The next morning, he brought her coffee in bed... and made love to her like it was the first time.

These women didn't beg. They didn't plead. They didn't even speak.

They transmitted.

And the men responded—not to the words, but to the feeling.

That's what this book has given you.

Now let's talk about what happens... if he doesn't respond.

If You Don't See Results Right Away

It doesn't mean your energy wasn't felt. It means the ripple hasn't hit the surface yet.

Every soul moves at their own pace.

Some are wide open.

Some have walls up.

Some are stubborn as hell.

But your energy always lands.

It's there, stirring under the surface, waking up old longings, making him restless in ways he doesn't even understand.

And the more you trust it—the faster it grows.

That's why I always recommend using guided meditations when you want to supercharge the technique even more.

➜ Guided audios allow your mind to sink naturally into the alpha state—the relaxed, dreamy state where you connect effortlessly.

➜ They keep you out of overthinking, self-doubt, and energy sabotage.

➜ They program the emotions and images into your subconscious automatically—while you relax and listen.

If you want to experience it even deeper, I've created a collection of special guided meditations designed exactly for this book.

You can check them out at http://laniestevens.com/. They're the perfect companion to everything you've learned in this book.

Remember: When you're playful, trusting, and powerful—your results multiply like wildfire.

Energy responds to certainty.

So claim it.

Own it.

And know: He already feels you. Whether he acts on it today, tomorrow, or six months from now—the bond has already been formed.

And it's not going anywhere.

Chapter 12: Q&A + Final Energy Check-In

Your Questions Answered, Your Power Reclaimed

Q: What if I'm the one who gets too attached?

A: Then it's time to check in with your energy.

This method is powerful—so powerful, in fact, that it can stir up intense feelings not just in *him*, but in *you*. That's part of the magic.

You're opening up the emotional, sensual, spiritual connection between two people. Of course you're going to feel something.

But if you find yourself obsessing, replaying, overdoing it, or spiraling into anxious attachment.

Pause.

Breathe.

Pull your energy back.

You are not powerless.

You are not waiting for crumbs.

You are the one sending the signal—not begging for a return text.

And the beauty of this method? You can redirect the power *any time*.

Seduce someone else.

Channel the energy into your art, your glow-up, your business.

Send it toward your future self—the woman who already has the love, devotion, and desire she craves.

This method doesn't make you clingy.

It makes you conscious.

And that's everything.

***

Q: Can I use this to get him back if he's with someone else?

A: You can—and many women have.

But here's the nuance: You're not "stealing" anyone. You're simply reconnecting a bond that already existed.

You're igniting a desire that may have gone dormant. You're whispering to his soul, not screaming at his ego. This isn't manipulation.

This is magnetism.

And if the relationship he's in now isn't energetically aligned, your presence—your essence—will stir something in him that feels missing.

One woman I know used this technique on a man who'd moved on, moved states, and moved in with someone else. She didn't go berserk. She didn't chase. She simply tapped in nightly with pure sexual energy, emotional memory, and intentional focus.

Within weeks he was calling. Within months he moved back. They're now planning their wedding.

Does it always play out like that? No.

But can it? Yes, queen.

Q: What if he ghosted me—or blocked me?

A: That just means you have a clean energy line.

When someone blocks you in the physical world, it's usually because they're overwhelmed, emotionally avoidant, or trying to shut down the connection.

But here's what most people don't realize:

Blocking someone on a phone doesn't block *energy*.

Practice Journal: Energetic Check-In

Before you close this chapter, take a moment to reflect on what this book has opened up inside you. This method wasn't just about reaching *him*. It was about reconnecting with *you*.

Ask yourself:

- Who have I been energetically connecting to—and why?
- How do I feel before, during, and after these sessions?
- What signs, dreams, or synchronicities have shown up since I began?
- Am I leading from confidence... or chasing from fear?
- What kind of love, sex, or connection do I now know I deserve?

Let your answers rise without judgment. You're not doing this to be perfect—you're doing it to be *powerful*.

The more you own your energy, the more magnetic you become.

And now... the signal is yours to send.

Thank You

If you've made it to the end of this book, I want to say one thing:

Thank you—and welcome. You've just stepped into a secret world most people never discover.

A world where feminine energy isn't passive—it's electric.

A world where thoughts shape desire, emotions seduce the mind, and connection can happen from miles away.

This isn't just a book. It's an activation.

You've remembered who you are—and what you can do.

Whether you were here to call back a lover, ignite new obsession, or just finally feel like the powerful, sensual woman you've always been deep down... I'm honored you let me be part of your journey.

And trust me—this is only the beginning.

You now know how to influence anyone with nothing but your energy.

So go play. Go experiment.

Go take everything you've just learned and make it your own.

And if you want more tools, meditations, secret rituals, or personal readings—come find me.

I'm always adding new magic. With fire, power, and so much love,

About the Author

Lanie Stevens—a bestselling author, energy influence expert, and creator of powerful feminine techniques that help women manifest love, command desire, and attract deep emotional connection—without chasing.

My signature methods combine subconscious reprogramming, quantum energy, emotional alchemy, and intuitive seduction. Thousands of women around the world have used these teachings to call back lovers, repair broken relationships, and unlock irresistible confidence from within.

My work goes beyond traditional dating and relationship advice. I teach women how to become magnetic on an energetic level—reaching a man's subconscious mind, bypassing logic, and planting emotional imprints that last.

To dive deeper into my secret techniques, visit:

http://laniestevens.com

The audiobook version available **ONLY** on my website. You'll also find exclusive meditations, audio programs, and life-changing tools to manifest love, confidence, and personal power.

Watch my YouTube channel here:

https://www.youtube.com/lanie-stevens

Explore The Love Goddess Series:

- Pussy Whip – Become the ultimate love goddess
- Pussy Whip 2 – Make your man behave the way you want
- How to Make Him Burn With Desire – Send him into a love trance
- Manifesting Love – Be the love magnet you were meant to be
- Fu*k the Rules – Break every dating rule they told you
- Breakup to Makeup – Get your ex back and keep him
- The Miracle Mindset – Make the impossible possible
- A Magical Love Spell – The ultimate love potion
- Positive Affirmations – Rewrite your reality with words
- Quantum Leaping – Rewire your mind and shift your identity
- Texting & Sexting – The key to igniting your relationship.